The Slowcooker Guide to the Keto Diet

100 Wholesome Delicious Keto Friendly Recipes

Additionally, the information found on the following pages is intended for informational purposes only and should thus be considered, universal. As befitting its nature, the information presented is without assurance regarding its continued validity or interim quality. Trademarks that mentioned are done without written consent and can in no way be considered an endorsement from the trademark holder.

Table of Contents

Introduction

Hello and thank you so much for your purchase of *The slowcooker Guide to the Keto Diet: 100 Wholesome Delicious Keto Friendly Recipes.*

In today's world, it is stressful to step on the scale and read the numbers our bodies produce. Yet, why aren't we more motivated to lessen what the scale tells us? While I do not recommend developing that a negative habit with your scale, I am here to provide you with a book that I believe can help a large population of folks who are unsure where to begin in their journey to better health.

I am sure you have heard of the ketogenic diet; this diet has many reputations, ranging from beneficial to unfavorable. It shakes up everything we know about giving our body the nutrition it needs for us to conquer everyday life.

Before you become prematurely disappointed and assume this is another book that tries its hardest to convince you to undergo the ketogenic diet, let me reassure you that this cookbook is not like that at all! This particular ketogenic cookbook gives readers a goldmine of value and allows them to determine the pros and cons of the ketogenic in their personal life before taking the plunge.

There is no diet out there that works for everyone, but you will never know how certain diets work unless you *try* them out! This book is also unique with what the ketogenic is paired with. The slowcooker is a highly underrated kitchen appliance that provides both singles and large families with the ability to dump ingredients, set the gadget, and let it do its magic as they continue to provide value to the world!

So, are you ready to dive into the keto slowcooker book? I hope you are! All you readers are in for an eye-opening treat. Every effort was made to ensure it is full of as much useful information as possible, please enjoy!

Chapter 1:
What is the Keto Diet?

Before we dive into the delicious recipes that this cookbook offers, it is a good idea to get a clear sense of the mission that the ketogenic diet offers those that undergo its power!

The Ketogenic Diet is based around a large consumption of fats, paired with the decrease of one's intake of carbohydrates. As you can imagine, this is why the keto diet is a magnificent tool for weight loss. But unlike other low-carb diets, the ketogenic is drastically different since it works in creating a sense of ketosis within the body.

Ketosis is a state where your body is metabolic, meaning that instead of using the power of carbohydrates for fuel, the body switches to the use of ketones instead as its main source of juice. Ketones are made from fat, which is a much more stable energy source than glucose ever will be. It takes about three to seven days of undergoing the ketogenic diet for your body to switch to a ketone fuel system. Since your body is using ketones as its food instead of glucose, it aids in shedding unwanted pounds of fat at a drastically quicker rate.

Foods to Enjoy on the Keto
- Meats:
  - BACON
  - Chicken
  - Ham
  - Red meats
  - Sausage

  - o Steak
  - o Turkey
  - o Etc.

- Fatty fishes:
  - o Salmon
  - o Trout
  - o Tuna
  - o etc.

- Eggs:
  - o omega-3
  - o whole
  - o etc.

- Butters and creams:
  - o "grass-fed" options are best

- Cheeses:
  - o any unprocessed cheeses
    - ▪ cheddar
    - ▪ cream cheese
    - ▪ Goat
    - ▪ mozzarella
    - ▪ etc.

- Nuts and seeds:
  - o Almonds
  - o chia seeds
  - o Flaxseeds
  - o pumpkin seeds
  - o Walnuts
  - o etc.

- Healthy oils:
    - avocado
    - coconut
    - extra-virgin
    - etc.

- Avocados

- Low carb veggies:
    - dark leafy greens
    - onions
    - peppers
    - tomatoes
    - etc.

Chapter 2:
The Ketogenic Benefits

The ketogenic diet is really beginning to gain traction in the world of better health among the population. The consumption of large amounts of carbohydrates for fuel can be potentially dangerous and aid in the development of negative health issues later down the road. This is why the bad rap that the consumption of fats once had is decreasing, all thanks to people's results from undergoing the keto diet!

The landscape of nutrition is always going to change, especially with the evolution of diets low in carbs. With so many folks becoming addicted to the intake of carbs and excess sugars in the day to day life, the ketogenic diet may be one of the best choices you make for yourself regarding your health and your overall longevity.

Benefits of the Keto Diet

Now that you have gotten a decent peek of what the ketogenic diet is all about, here is a list of amazing health benefits that have the power to convince just about anyone to rethink what this particular diet can do for your health!

- Daily benefits include:

  o Longer periods of time feeling satisfied and not dwelling on weird cravings.

  o Reduction in temptations that lead to bad choices of fuel.

- o Energy levels stay consistently high throughout the day.

- Capability to lose more weight at a faster rate

- Ability to maintain optimal cholesterol levels

- Decrease in blood sugar levels, which prevents and reverses diabetes

- Decrease in overall appetite

- Decrease in negative triglyceride levels

- Decrease in development of heart disease and experiencing a stroke

- Decrease in high blood pressure levels

Chapter 3:
The Past Behind the Keto

The idea of fasting and sticking to other dietary regimens have been used since way before our time, at least since 500 B.C. In fact, this type of body fueling was studied in great detail by Greek and Indian physicians.

The first real and well document scientific study of the keto diet was made by France in the year 1911. In the epileptic world, potassium bromide was being used as a form of treatment but had negative side effects regarding the patients' mental health and mental capabilities. It was then that patients underwent low calorie and vegan diets, combined with a dose of fasting. This was when patients began to show real improvement!

The idea behind the ketogenic diet was utilized to mimic the metabolism when fasting to treat folks with epilepsy. It wasn't until the 1920's that modern physicians began using the idea of the ketogenic diet for more than just an epilepsy treatment. This therapy at the time was only used in a small number of hospitals that centered their services on children's health.

In the 1960's, ketones were shown to produce much more energy than that of a diet filled with carbohydrates. In 1971, a physician named Peter Huttenlocher finally created the ketogenic diet as it is known today, which centered around the reduction of calories that came from carbs by sixty-percent.

Over the past fifteen years, the ketogenic diet has exploded into more than a scientific kind of diet and has become one of the most effective treatments known to the human race in a fight against children and adults with epilepsy issues. In today's world, it is known by some as merely a diet fad, while hundreds of thousands of others have utilized the keto diet to drastically change their lives in positive ways.

Chapter 4:
Side Effects of the Keto Diet

While the ketogenic diet is very healthy in nature, there are drastic side effects that newbies of this diet need to be aware of before starting the process. Thankfully, these and many side effects while on the ketogenic only occur during the beginning process of undergoing the diet, when your body is adapting to its new source of fuel.

Side Effects on the Ketogenic

This is a list of the most common side effects you may experience when you begin your transition from your everyday diet that your body has been using to that of using fats as fuel:

- Decrease in strength
- Decrease in ability to perform physically
- Heart palpitations
- Bad breathe, caused by the rise in ketone levels
- Problems sleeping soundly
- Flu-like symptoms
- Cravings for sugar
- Muscle cramps
- Dizziness
- Drowsiness
- The need to frequently urinate

- Diarrhea

- Constipation

- Hypoglycemia

The three main reasons for these types of symptoms when beginning your keto journey are due to:

1. Mineral and electrolyte deficiencies

2. Low blood sugar

3. HPA, or hypothalamic pituitary adrenal dysfunction

While the three causes are different, they all relate to one another regarding the ketogenic diet. Your body has been used to running on sugar for years, so when you switch its source of fuel to that of fats, your body needs to be given the time to build the cellular structures necessary to generate and use fats.

The 'Keto Flu'

This is probably one of the worst side effects of undergoing the keto diet and is well-known in the ketogenic world as the 'keto flu.' This occurs when people start out on this diet and experience very low levels of sodium and electrolytes in their bodies. Symptoms include:

- Fatigue

- Headaches

- Cough

- Sniffling

- Irritability

- Nausea and vomiting

This is not near as terrible as the real flu that everyone avoids, but still can make you feel pretty crumby and wonder why you underwent this diet in the first place. Don't give up hope! It takes a few days to a week to allow your body to switch its source of fuel and adapt to the changes. Just be prepared to not feel your best during this time and limit your overall activity levels.

So, why does the keto flu occur? Simple because dieters are eliminating processed foods and consuming whole, natural foods. This can cause a major drop in sodium consumption.

Stopping the 'Keto Flu'

There are some things you can do to prepare your body for the transition from carbs to fats as a fuel source. The best way is to simply add more sodium and sources of electrolytes into your system.

- Add more salt to the food you devour

- Drink natural broths, such as bone broth

- Consume foods high in sodium, such as bacon and pickled vegetables

Chapter 5:
Veggie and Vegan Recipes

Stuffed Eggplant

Calories: 180 Carbs: 2g Fat: 13g Protein: 9g

Servings: 6

Cooking: 1 ½ hours

Ingredients:

- 1 seeded and chopped green bell pepper
- 1 tbsp. tomato paste
- 1 tsp. cumin
- 1 tsp. raw coconut sugar
- 2 chopped red onions
- 3 tbsp. chopped parsley
- 4 chopped tomatoes
- 4 minced garlic cloves
- 4 tbsp. olive oil
- 6 eggplants

Preparation:

1. Remove eggplant skins with a vegetable peeler. Slice eggplants lengthwise and sprinkle with salt. Allow to sit half an hour to sweat.

2. Place eggplants into the slowcooker. Cook on high 20 minutes.

3. Sauté onions in a heated pan with olive oil. Stir bell pepper and garlic with onions and sauté for an additional 1 to 2 minutes.

4. Pour mixture into eggplants into the slowcooker. Cook 20 minutes on high.

5. Season with pepper and salt and add parsley, tomato paste, cumin, sugar, and tomato. Cook another 10 minutes, stir well and serve!

Bacon Cheddar Broccoli Salad

Calories: 189 Carbs: 8g Fat: 21g Protein: 8g

Servings: 15

Cooking: 2 hours

Ingredients:

Dressing:

- ¼ C. sweetener of choice
- 1 C. keto mayo
- 2 tbsp. organic vinegar

Broccoli Salad:

- ½ diced red onion
- 4 ounces cheddar cheese
- ½ pound bacon, cooked and chopped
- 1 large head broccoli
- 1/8 C. sunflower seeds
- 1/8 C. pumpkin seeds

Preparation:

- For the dressing, whisk all dressing components together, adjusting taste pepper and salt and add to your slowcooker.

- Set pot to low to cook for a couple hours till cheese is melted and everything is combined.

- Serve warm!

Cracked-Out Keto Slaw

Calories: 360 Carbs: 5g Fat: 33g Protein: 7g

Servings: 2

Cooking: 1 ¾ hours

Ingredients:

- ½ C. chopped macadamia nuts
- 1 tbsp. sesame oil
- 1 tsp. chili paste
- 1 tsp. vinegar
- 2 garlic cloves
- 2 tbsp. tamari
- 4 C. shredded cabbage

Preparation:

1. Toss cabbage with chili paste, sesame oil, vinegar, and tamari. Add to slowcooker.

2. Add minced garlic and mix well.

3. Set to cook on high 1 ½ hours.

4. Stir in macadamia nuts. Cook 5 minutes more.

5. Garnish with sesame seeds before serving.

Zucchini Pasta

Calories: 181 Carbs: 6g Fat: 13g Protein: 5g

Servings: 4

Cooking: 1-2 hours

Ingredients:

- ¼ C. olive oil
- ½ C. basil
- ½ tsp. red pepper flakes
- 1-pint halved cherry tomatoes
- 1 sliced red onion
- 2 pounds spiralized zucchini
- 4 minced garlic cloves

Preparation:

1. Sauté onion and garlic 3 minutes till fragrant in olive oil.

2. Add zucchini noodles to slowcooker and season with pepper and salt. Cook 60 minutes on high heat.

3. Mix in tomatoes, basil, onion, garlic, and red pepper. Cook another 20 minutes.

4. Add parmesan cheese to slowcooker. Mix thoroughly and cook 10 minutes to melt cheese. Devour!

Twice Baked Spaghetti Squash

Calories: 230 Carbs: 4g Fat: 17g Protein: 12g

Servings: 4

Cooking: 6 hours

Ingredients:

- ¼ tsp. pepper
- ¼ tsp. salt
- ½ C. grated parmesan cheese
- 1 tsp. oregano
- 2 minced garlic cloves
- 2 small spaghetti squashes
- 2 tbsp. butter
- 4 slices Provolone cheese

Preparation:

1. Cut spaghetti squash in half lengthwise, discarding innards. Set gently into your pot.

2. Cook on high heat for 4 hours.

3. Take squash innards and mix with parmesan cheese and butter. Then mix in pepper, salt, garlic, and oregano.

4. Add squash innards mixture to the middle of cooked squash halves.

5. Cook on high for another 1-2 hours till middles are deliciously bubbly.

Mushroom Risotto

Calories: 438 Carbs: 5g Fat: 17g Protein: 12g

Servings: 4

Cooking: 3-4 hours

Ingredients:

- ¼ C. vegetable broth
- 1-pound sliced Portobello mushrooms
- 1-pound sliced white mushrooms
- 1/3 C. grated parmesan cheese
- 2 diced shallots
- 3 tbsp. chopped chives
- 3 tbsp. coconut oil
- 4 ½ C. riced cauliflower
- 4 tbsp. butter

Preparation:

1. Heat up oil and sauté mushrooms 3 minutes till soft. Discard liquid and set to the side.

2. Add oil to skillet and sauté shallots 60 seconds.

3. Pour all recipe components into your pot and mix well to combine.

4. Cook 3 hours on high heat.

5. Serve topped with parmesan cheese.

Vegan Bibimbap

Calories: 119 Carbs: 0g Fat: 18g Protein: 8g

Servings: 4

Cooking: 45 minutes

Ingredients:

- ½ cucumber, sliced into strips
- 1 grated carrot
- 1 sliced red bell pepper
- 1 tbsp. soy sauce
- 1 tsp. sesame oil
- 10-ounces riced cauliflower
- 2 tbsp. rice vinegar
- 2 tbsp. sesame seeds
- 2 tbsp. sriracha sauce
- 4-5 broccoli florets
- 7-ounces tempeh, sliced into squares
- Liquid sweetener

Preparation:

1. In a bowl, combine tempeh squares with 1 tbsp. soy sauce and 2 tbsp. vinegar. Set aside to soak. Slice veggies.

2. Add carrot, broccoli, and peppers to slowcooker. Cook on high 30 minutes.

3. Add cauliflower rice to the pot, cook 5 minutes.

4. Add sweetener, oil, soy sauce, vinegar, and sriracha to slowcooker. Don't hesitate to add a bit of water if you find the mixture to be too thick.

Avocado Pesto Kelp Noodles

Calories: 321 Carbs: 1g Fat: 32g Protein: 2g

Servings: 2

Cooking: 1 ½ hours

Ingredients:

Pesto:

- ¼ C. basil
- ½ C. extra-virgin olive oil
- 1 avocado
- 1 C. baby spinach leaves
- 1 tsp. salt
- 1-2 garlic cloves
- 1 package of kelp noodles

Preparation:

1. Add kelp noodles to slowcooker with just enough water to cover them. Cook on high 45-60 minutes.

2. In the meantime, combine pesto ingredients in a blender, blending till smooth and incorporated.

3. Stir in pesto and heat noodle mixture 10 minutes.

Vegan Cream of Mushroom Soup

Calories: 281 Carbs: 3g Fat: 16g Protein: 11g

Servings: 2

Cooking: 1 ¾ hours

Ingredients:

- ¼ tsp. sea salt
- ½ diced yellow onion
- ½ tsp. extra-virgin olive oil
- 1 ½ C. diced white mushrooms
- 1 2/3 C. unsweetened almond milk
- 1 tsp. onion powder
- 2 C. cauliflower florets

Preparation:

1. Add cauliflower, pepper, salt, onion powder, and milk to slowcooker. Stir and set to cook on high 1 hour.

2. With olive oil, sauté onions and mushrooms together 8 to 10 minutes till softened.

3. Allow cauliflower mixture to cool off a bit and add to blender. Blend until smooth. Then blend in mushroom mixture.

4. Pour back into slowcooker and heat 30 minutes.

Creamy Curry Sauce Noodle Bowl

Calories: 110 Carbs: 1g Fat: 9g Protein: 7g

Servings: 4

Cooking: 1-2 hours

Ingredients:

- ½ head chopped cauliflower
- 1 diced red bell pepper
- 1 pack of Kanten Noodles
- 2 chopped carrots
- 2 handfuls of mixed greens
- Chopped cilantro

Curry Sauce:

- ¼ C. avocado oil mayo
- ¼ C. water
- ¼ tsp./ ginger
- ½ tsp. pepper
- 1 ½ tsp. coriander
- 1 tsp. cumin
- 1 tsp turmeric
- 2 tbsp. apple cider vinegar
- 2 tbsp. avocado oil
- 2 tsp. curry powder

Diet *Preparation:*

1. Add all ingredients, minus curry sauce components, to your slowcooker. Set to cook on high 1-2 hours.

2. In the meantime, add all of curry sauce ingredients to a blender. Puree until smooth.

3. Pour over veggie and noodle mixture. Stir well to coat.

Spinach Artichoke Casserole

Calories: 141 Carbs: 7g Fat: 9g Protein: 10g

Servings: 10

Cooking: 4-6 hours

Ingredients:

- ½ tsp. pepper
- ¾ C. coconut flour
- ¾ C. unsweetened almond milk
- 1 C. grated parmesan cheese
- 1 tbsp. baking powder
- 1 tsp. salt
- 3 minced garlic cloves
- 5-ounces chopped spinach
- 6-ounces chopped artichoke hearts
- 8 eggs

Preparation:

1. Grease the inside of your slowcooker.

2. Whisk ½ of parmesan cheese, pepper, salt, garlic, artichoke hearts, spinach, eggs, and almond milk together.

3. Add baking powder and coconut flour, combining well.

4. Spread into the slowcooker. Sprinkle with remaining parmesan cheese.

5. Cook 2 to 3 hours on high or you can cook 4 to 6 hours on a lower heat setting.

Chapter 6:
Soups and Stews

Jalapeno Popper Chicken Soup

Calories: 289 Carbs: 6g Fat: 20g Protein: 14g

Servings: 6

Cooking: 3-4 hours

Ingredients:

- ¼ chopped onion
- ½ pound bacon
- 1 C. water
- 1 can cream of chicken soup
- 1 chopped jalapeno pepper
- 1 tsp. pepper
- 1 tsp. salt
- 2 cans of white great northern beans
- 2 seeded/chopped jalapeno peppers
- 2 tbsp. taco seasoning
- 3 boneless chicken breasts
- 8 ounces cream cheese

Preparation:

1. Put chicken in the bottom of slowcooker. Sprinkle with taco seasoning, pepper, and salt. Then add water, cream of chicken soup, beans, onions, and jalapenos. Stir well to incorporate.

2. Cook on high 3-4 hours or opt to cook on low 6 to 8 hours.

3. Shred chicken and add back to pot.

4. Cube cream cheese and stir into soup till it melts.

5. Fry bacon, chop it up and add to soup.

6. Serve with additional bacon, jalapeno peppers, cheddar cheese, sour cream, etc.

Green Chili Enchilada Soup

Calories: 278 Carbs: 5g Fat: 19g Protein: 11g

Servings: 8

Cooking: 7 hours

Ingredients:

- ¾ C. water
- 1 tsp. garlic powder
- 1 tsp. onion powder
- 15-ounce jar salsa
- 2 tbsp. cumin
- 24-ounces chicken breasts
- 32-ounces chicken broth
- 4-ounce can diced green chilies
- 8-ounces softened cream cheese

Preparation:

1. Put chicken in the bottom of slowcooker. Add all seasoning and herbs to chicken, mixing well to incorporate.

2. Set to cook on low 7 hours.

3. Mix in cream cheese, stirring till dissolved. Cook an additional half an hour to heat soup.

Chicken Stew

Calories: 228 Carbs: 6g Fat: 11g Protein: 23g

Servings: 4

Cooking: 4 hours

Ingredients:

- ¼ tsp. dried thyme
- ½ C. heavy cream
- ½ C. peeled and diced carrots
- ½ tsp. dried oregano
- 1 C. diced celery
- 1 C. spinach
- 1 sprig rosemary
- 2 C. chicken stock
- 28-ounces skinless, deboned chicken thighs, sliced into 1-inch pieces

Preparation:

1. Add oregano, thyme, garlic, rosemary, chicken thighs, onion, celery, carrots, and chicken stock to your slowcooker.

2. Cook on high 2 hours or cook on low 4 hours.

3. Stir spinach and heavy cream into mixture.

4. Whisk 10 minutes till it becomes a bit thicker.

Tip! You can use a bit of xanthan gum to help stew thicken more.

Autumn Beef and Veggie Stew

Calories: 553 Carbs: 9g Fat: 39g Protein: 31g

Servings: 8-10

Cooking: 6 hours

Ingredients:

- ½ C. ghee
- 1 ½ tsp. salt
- 1 C. vegetable stock
- 1 rutabaga
- 1 tbsp. paprika
- 1 tsp. chili powder
- 1 tsp. coriander seeds
- 1 tsp. ginger
- 1 tsp. turmeric powder
- 1 white onion
- 14-ounce can chopped tomatoes
- 2 bay leaves
- 2 cinnamon sticks
- 2 tbsp. cumin
- 3 ½ pounds boneless braising steaks
- 4 garlic cloves
- 4-5 zucchinis

Preparation:

1. Turn slowcooker to high.

2. Pat down steaks and season with pepper and salt.

3. Place steaks into a skillet with ¼ cup of ghee. Sear till just browned lightly. Place into the slowcooker.

4. Peel and dice garlic and onion. Put into a pan with ghee that remains, sautéing till fragrant.

5. Add turmeric, coriander, chili powder, ginger, cumin, broth, paprika, and tomatoes to pot. Then add bay leaves and cinnamon sticks.

6. Set to cook on high 3 hours.

7. Push meat to one side of the pot.

8. Peel and dice rutabaga and add to slowcooker.

9. Add rutabaga to other side. Cook another 60 minutes

10. Dice zucchini. Add zucchini to the same side as rutabaga and mix well to combine with cooking juices.

11. Discard bay leaves and cinnamon sticks.

12. Cook another 2 hours. Once zucchini and rutabaga are tender to the touch of a fork, the stew is done!

Bacon Cabbage Chuck Beef Stew

Calories: 378 Carbs: 4g Fat: 24g Protein: 28g

Servings: 5

Cooking: 7 hours

Ingredients:

- ½ pound uncured bacon, sliced into strips
- 1 C. beef bone broth
- 1 head of cabbage
- 1 peeled and smashed the garlic clove
- 1 sprig thyme
- 2 peeled and sliced red onions
- 2-3 pounds chuck roast

Preparation:

1. Place slices of bacon into the bottom of slowcooker.

2. Slice chuck roast into bite-sized pieces.

3. Add garlic and onion slices to bacon.

4. Add roast on top of onion and garlic.

5. Then add cabbage slices along with thyme, broth, and a few pinches of pepper and sea salt.

6. Set to cook on low 7 hours.

Chunky Beef and Cauliflower Stew

Calories: 413 Carbs: 9g Fat: 39g Protein: 31g

Servings: 4

Cooking: 5 hours

Ingredients:

- ½ C. dry white wine
- ½ tsp. pepper
- 1 ¼ pounds beef sirloin tip roast
- 1 bay leaf
- 1 onion
- 1-pound of cauliflower
- 1 tsp. olive oil
- 1 tsp. thyme
- 2 ½ C. beef stock
- 2 tbsp. tomato paste
- 3 celery stalks
- 3 minced garlic cloves
- 3 tbsp. all-purpose flour
- 4 chopped carrots
- 4-ounce can of mushrooms

Diet *Preparation:*

1. Warm up some olive oil in a skillet and proceed to sear beef cubes.

2. Cut up the head of cauliflower into small pieces.

3. Chop up onion and celery into smaller pieces as well.

4. Sauté carrots and onions in beef grease 10 minutes till golden.

5. With white wine, deglaze the pan, getting cooking bits from the bottom.

6. Add meat, carrots, onions, cooking bit and remaining ingredients to your slowcooker. Stir well to incorporate.

7. Cook for 5 hours on low or 3 hours on high.

Double Beef Stew

Calories: 222 Carbs: 11g Fat: 7g Protein: 27g

Servings: 6

Cooking: 2 hours

Ingredients:

- 1 C. beef broth
- 1 tbsp. chili mix
- 1 tbsp. Worcestershire sauce
- 2 14.5-ounce cans diced tomatoes
- 2 tsp. hot sauce
- 5-pounds beef stew meat

Preparation:

1. Set slowcooker to high.

2. Pour all ingredients into the pot and stir well to combine.

3. Set to cook 6 hours on high.

4. Break up meat and pull apart with a fork.

5. Season if needed.

6. Set to cook 2 hours on low. Devour!

Beef and Sweet Potato Stew

Calories: 396 Carbs: 6g Fat: 29g Protein: 21g

Servings: 8

Cooking: 4-6 hours

Ingredients:

- ½ - 1 tsp. salt
- ½ tsp. pepper
- 1 ½ C. beef broth
- 1 crushed beef bouillon cube
- 1 sweet potato
- 1 tsp. paprika
- 1/3 C. all-purpose flour
- 10-ounce halved baby potatoes
- 14-ounce can diced tomatoes
- 2 bay leaves
- 2 sliced carrots
- 3 pounds beef stew meat
- 4 crushed garlic cloves
- 4 tbsp. chopped parsley

Preparation:

1. Pour flour and stew meat into slowcooker. Stir well to coat meat.

2. Add remaining ingredients to the pot, minus parsley and bay leaves. Stir well to incorporate thoroughly. Add bay leaves to the top.

3. Cook 8-10 hours on low or 4-6 hours on high.

4. Season with pepper and salt, discard bay leaves.

5. Serve garnished with parsley.

Lasagna Soup

Calories: 391 Carbs: 2g Fat: 25g Protein: 18g

Servings: 8

Cooking: 2 hours

Ingredients:

- ½ C. heavy whipping cream
- ½ C. shredded parmesan cheese
- 1 C. cottage cheese
- 1 C. shredded mozzarella cheese
- 1 diced sweet onion
- 1 tbsp. Italian blend herbs
- 1 tbsp. Italian sausage seasoning
- 1 tsp. garlic salt
- 1 tsp. paprika
- 2 14.5-ounce cans fire roasted tomatoes
- 2 C. beef broth
- 2 diced garlic cloves
- 2-pound ground pork
- 2 tsp. red pepper flakes
- 5-6 basil leaves

Preparation:

1. Pour seasonings, tomatoes, garlic, onion, and meat into slowcooker. Set to cook on high 2 hours.

2. Break up meat.

3. Add cottage cheese to a blender, blending till liquefied. Add to soup.

4. Set to low till you are ready to devour!

Pizza Soup

Calories: 405 Carbs: 4g Fat: 31g Protein: 18g

Servings: 8

Cooking: 4-5 hours

Ingredients:

- 1 C. mini pepperonis
- 1 C. water
- 1 tbsp. Italian seasoning
- 1-2 pounds browned ground sausage
- 14.5-ounce can beef broth
- 16-ounces cream cheese
- 2 C. marinara sauce
- 2.25-ounce can black olives, drained
- 4 ounces mushrooms

Preparation:

1. Within your slowcooker, combine all ingredients till well incorporated.

2. Cook 2-3 hours on high or 4-5 hours on low.

3. Serve topped with mozzarella cheese if you so choose.

Bacon Cheeseburger Soup

Calories: 359 Carbs: 4g Fat: 16g Protein: 21g

Servings: 8

Cooking: 1 hour

Ingredients:

- ½ C. heavy cream
- ½ tsp. garlic powder
- ½ tsp. ground red pepper
- ½ tsp. onion powder
- ½ tsp. pepper
- 1 C. shredded cheddar cheese
- 1 tsp. chili powder
- 1 tsp. cumin
- 12 ounces ground beef
- 2 ½ tbsp. tomato paste
- 2 tbsp. butter
- 2 tbsp. yellow mustard
- 3 C. beef broth
- 3 diced dill pickles
- 3-ounces cream cheese
- 5 slices of bacon

Preparation:

1. Cook bacon. Take out of pan and brown beef in the same pan in bacon grease.

2. Add spices and butter to another pan. Cook 45 seconds. Add cream cheese, mustard, cheese, tomato paste, and broth to butter and spice mixture. Cook 5 minutes to melt cream cheese.

3. Add pickles and heavy cream to the sauce.

4. Pour sauce over meat and simmer 5-10 minutes.

5. Pour everything into your slowcooker. Set to cook on high 1 hour.

Chapter 7:
Chili Recipes

Bacon Chili

Calories: 527 Carbs: 7g Fat: 37g Protein: 51g

Servings: 5

Cooking: 5 hours

Ingredients:

- ½ tsp. pepper
- ¾ white onion
- 1 green bell pepper
- 1 Roma tomato
- 1 tbsp. chili powder
- 1 tsp. Worcestershire sauce
- 1 tsp. oregano
- 1 tsp. salt
- 2 C. chicken stock
- 2 jalapeno peppers
- 2 tsp. cumin
- 3 garlic cloves
- 30-ounces lean ground beef
- 5 slices of bacon

Preparation:

1. Chop up bacon and add to pan. Cook till fat renders out and bacon is almost cooked. Then add beef to pan, cooking till some color forms.

2. Chop up jalapeno peppers and garlic finely. Roughly chop up onion, bell pepper, and tomato.

3. Add 2 cups of stock to slowcooker along with all other ingredients. Combine well.

4. Cook 5 hours on low or 2 ½ hours on high.

Steak Lover's Chili

Calories: 198 Carbs: 6g Fat: 19g Protein: 11g

Servings: 8

Cooking: 6 hours

Ingredients:

- ¼ tsp. cayenne pepper
- ½ C. sliced leeks
- ½ tsp. cumin
- ½ tsp. salt
- 1 C. chicken stock
- 1 tbsp. chili powder
- 1/8 tsp. pepper
- 2 ½ pounds steak, sliced into 1-inch cubes
- 2 C. canned tomatoes

Optional Toppings:

- ¼ C. shredded cheddar cheese
- ½ sliced avocado
- 1 tsp. cilantro
- 2 tbsp. sour cream

Preparation:

1. Pour all ingredients into your slow cooker, except topping components.

2. Stir well to incorporate. Set to cook on high 6 hours.

3. Shred cubes of steak and break up tomatoes.

4. Serve topped with desired toppings.

Buffalo Chicken Chili

Calories: 277 Carbs: 11g Fat: 14g Protein: 17g

Servings: 8

Cooking: 8 hours

Ingredients:

- ¼ - ½ C. buffalo wing sauce
- ¼ tsp. salt
- ½ tsp. celery salt
- ½ tsp. dried cilantro
- ½ tsp. garlic powder
- ½ tsp. onion powder
- 1 C. frozen corn
- 1 package of ranch dressing mix
- 1-pound ground chicken
- 14.5-ounce can fire roasted tomatoes
- 15-ounce can white navy beans
- 2 C. chicken broth
- 8-ounces cream cheese

Preparation:

1. Brown chicken in skillet till cooked. Place into the slowcooker.

2. Mix in all remaining ingredients to chicken, mixing well to incorporate.

3. Cook 4 hours on high or 8 hours on low.

4. Stir well to incorporate cream cheese and wing sauce throughout chili mixture.

No Bean Chili

Calories: 201 Carbs: 2g Fat: 19g Protein: 21g

Servings: 6

Cooking: 6-7 hours

Ingredients:

- 1 C. water
- 1 packet of chili seasoning
- 14.5-ounce can diced tomatoes
- 14.5-ounce can tomato sauce
- 2 pounds lean ground beef

Preparation:

1. Cook ground beef and then add to slowcooker.

2. Add the rest of your ingredients, stirring thoroughly to combine well.

3. Cook on low heat 6-7 hours.

4. Serve topped with favorite toppings such as sour cream, cheese, diced onion, etc.

Kickin' Chili

Calories: 137 Carbs: 5g Fat: 15g Protein: 16g

Servings: 6

Cooking: 6-8 hours

Ingredients:

- ¼ C. pickled jalapeno slices
- ½ tsp. cayenne pepper
- 1 bay leaf
- 1 chopped red onion
- 1 tsp. garlic powder
- 1 tsp. onion powder
- 1 tsp. oregano
- 1 tsp. pepper
- 14.5-ounce can stewed tomatoes
- 14.5-ounce can tomatoes with green chilies
- 2 ½ pounds ground beef
- 2 tbsp. cumin
- 2 tbsp. Worcestershire sauce
- 2 tsp. salt
- 3 diced celery ribs
- 4 tbsp. chili powder
- 4 tbsp. minced garlic
- 6-ounce can tomato paste

Preparation:

1. Turn slowcooker to low.

2. Brown beef in skillet along with pepper, salt, and 2 tablespoons of minced garlic. Drain excess grease. Pour beef into the slowcooker.

3. Add remaining recipe components and mix well.

4. Cook 6-8 hours on low.

Creamy White Chicken Chili

Calories: 486 Carbs: 6g Fat: 33g Protein: 39g

Servings: 6

Cooking: 7 hours

Ingredients:

- ½ C. chicken stock
- ½ C. heavy cream
- ½ C. sour cream
- 1 tsp. cumin
- 1 tsp. garlic powder
- 2 pounds chicken
- 2 tsp. chili powder
- 3 tbsp. butter
- 4-ounces cream cheese
- 9-ounces chopped green chilies

Toppings:

- 1 C. shredded pepper jack cheese
- 1/3 C. peeled and chopped red onion
- 1/3 C. chopped cilantro

Preparation:

1. Place chicken in the slowcooker. Add green chilies, chicken stock, garlic powder, cumin, and chili powder to chicken.

2. Set to cook on low 7 hours.

3. 60 minutes before you plan to eat, heat sour cream, cream cheese, heavy cream, and butter together in a pan, stirring till smooth.

4. Shred chicken.

5. Pour cream cheese mixture over chicken, combining well to incorporate.

6. Sprinkle with pepper jack, red onion, and cilantro.

Old-Fashioned Low-Carb Slowcooker Chili

Calories: 318 Carbs: 4g Fat: 24g Protein: 17g

Servings: 8

Cooking: 3 hours

Ingredients:
- 1 ½ C. diced celery
- 1 C. beef broth
- 1 chopped yellow onion
- 1 tbsp. cumin
- 1 tsp. garlic powder
- 1 tsp. Italian seasoning
- 1 tsp. pepper
- 1 tsp. salt
- 14.5-ounce can crushed tomatoes
- 14.5-ounce can diced tomatoes with green chilies
- 2-pounds lean ground beef
- 2 tbsp. crushed red pepper flakes
- 3 tbsp. chili powder
- 3 tbsp. minced garlic
- 6-ounces tomato paste

Preparation:

1. Cook beef in a pan until browned and drain grease. Add garlic to pan and sauté 60 seconds.

2. Place beef in the slowcooker. Add remaining ingredients to beef.

3. Stir to combine well.

4. Cook 6 hours on low or 3 hours on high.

Secret Chocolate Chili

Calories: 492 Carbs: 7g Fat: 25g Protein: 17g

Servings: 4

Cooking: 4 hours

Ingredients:

- ½ onion
- 1 C. beef broth
- 1 C. black coffee
- 1 tbsp. chili powder
- 1 tbsp. cocoa powder
- 1 tbsp. soy sauce
- 1 tsp. cayenne pepper
- 1 tsp. cumin
- 10 drops liquid stevia
- 2 cans whole tomatoes
- 2-pounds ground beef
- 2 tbsp. butter
- 2 tbsp. Worcestershire sauce
- 2 tsp. garlic
- 2 tsp. paprika
- 6 slices of bacon
- 8-ounces kielbasa

Preparation:

1. Puree both cans of tomatoes in a food processor and add to slowcooker.

2. Add spices and all liquid ingredients minus garlic and butter to sauce in the slowcooker.

3. Add stevia.

4. Brown beef in a pan. Drain and put to the side.

5. Chop onion then sauté it in a pan until softened.

6. Add bacon and kielbasa to the pan with onion, cooking till bacon is crispy.

7. Add sausage and bacon mixture along with garlic powder to slowcooker.

8. Add beef to slowcooker.

9. Set to cook on high 4 hours.

Not Your Caveman's Chili

Calories: 390 Carbs: 5g Fat: 16g Protein: 27g

Servings: 4

Cooking: 3 ½ - 4 hours

Ingredients:

- 1 ½ tsp cumin
- 1 C. beef broth
- 1 green pepper
- 1 onion
- 1 tsp. cayenne pepper
- 1 tsp. oregano
- 1 tsp. pepper
- 1 tsp. salt
- 1 tsp. Worcestershire sauce
- 1/3 C. tomato paste
- 2 ½ tbsp. chili powder
- 2-pounds stew meat
- 2 tbsp. olive oil
- 2 tbsp. soy sauce
- 2 tsp. fish sauce
- 2 tsp. minced garlic
- 2 tsp. paprika

Preparation:

1. Chop up half of your meat into bite-sized pieces. Place the other half of your meat into your food processor, blending until ground.

2. Cut up onion and pepper into tiny pieces.

3. Mix all your spices together.

4. Sauté beef in the pan along with ground beef.

5. Sauté veggies in meat grease until fragrant

6. Add all ingredients into your slowcooker.

7. Simmer on high for 2 ½ hours. Stir and simmer 20-30 more minutes.

5-Ingredient Chili

Calories: 503 Carbs: 6g Fat: 41g Protein: 29g

Servings: 4

Cooking: 2-3 hours

Ingredients:

- 15-ounces tomato sauce
- 2 diced onions
- Cumin and other spices to achieve desired taste, such as cilantro, garlic, salt, chili powder, etc.
- 3-4 cans diced tomatoes
- 3-4 pounds meat of choice (ground turkey, bison, sausage, venison, beef, etc.)

Preparation:

1. Pour all ingredients into your slowcooker. Stir well to incorporate.

2. Cook 2-3 hours on high or 5-6 hours on low.

Chapter 8:
Poultry Recipes

Crack Chicken

Calories: 275 Carbs: 4g Fat: 14g Protein: 11g

Servings: 8

Cooking: 6-8 hours

Ingredients:

- ½-pound bacon, cooked and crumbled
- 1 packet of ranch dressing mix
- 1-pound boneless, skinless chicken breast
- 8-ounces cream cheese

Preparation:

1. Place dressing mix, cream cheese, and chicken into the slowcooker.

2. Cook 6-8 hours on low or 4 hours on high.

3. Shred meat with two forks and thoroughly mix with bacon. Enjoy!

Crispy slowcooker Chicken Thighs

Calories: 577 Carbs: 1g Fat: 43g Protein: 44g

Servings: 4-6

Cooking: 6-7 hours

Ingredients:

- ½ tsp. garlic powder
- ½ tsp. onion powder
- ¾ tsp. paprika
- 1 tsp. salt
- 6-8 bone-in, skin-on chicken thighs

Preparation:

1. Mix onion powder, garlic powder, salt, and paprika together.

2. Coat chicken thighs with seasoning mixture.

3. Place chicken into your slowcooker, skin side up.

4. Set to cook on low 6-7 hours until tender.

Mexican Turkey Loaf

Calories: 246 Carbs: 6g Fat: 13g Protein: 26g

Servings: 8-12

Cooking: 5-6 hours

Ingredients:

- 1 C. dried breadcrumbs
- 1 C. shredded cheese of choice
- 1 carrot
- 1 celery stalk
- 1 egg
- 1 onion
- 1-pound ground turkey
- 1 red bell pepper
- 1 taco seasoning packet
- 1/3 C. sour cream
- 19-ounce can enchilada sauce
- 4.5-ounce can chopped green chilies

Preparation:

1. In a big bowl, add both ground meats. Then add taco seasoning, sour cream, egg, and breadcrumbs.

2. Trim vegetables and dump into a food processor. Mix veggies till they turn out to be smooth. Dump veggie puree in a bowl.

3. With your hands, mix up ingredients till well incorporated. Then, shape mixture into a log and place into your slowcooker.

4. Pour enchilada sauce over the top.

5. Set to cook on low 5-6 hours.

6. Sprinkle with cheese right before serving.

Keto Chicken Tikka Masala

Calories 453 – Protein 26g – Carbs 7g – Fat 31g

Servings: 5

Cooking: 3 ½ hours

Ingredients:

- 1 ½ pounds bone-in chicken thighs
- 1 C. coconut milk
- 1 C. heavy cream
- 1-pound boneless skinless chicken thighs
- 1 tsp. guar gum
- 1" grated ginger root
- 10-ounce can diced tomatoes
- 2 tbsp. olive oil
- 2 tsp. Paprika
- 2 tsp. onion powder
- 3 minced cloves garlic
- 3 tbsp. tomato paste
- 4 tsp. salt
- 5 tsp. garam masala

Preparation:

1. De-bone the bone-in thighs. Cut chicken into pieces. Keep the skin on as much as you can.

2. Place chicken in the slowcooker. Grate ginger and sprinkle over the top.

3. Pour in all dry spices into the slowcooker. Combine well.

4. Mix in tomato paste, diced tomatoes, and olive oil, stirring well.

5. Add ½ cup coconut milk and mix.

6. Cook 3 hours on high or 6 hours on low.

7. When time is up, add remaining coconut milk along with guar gum and heavy cream. Mix thoroughly.

8. Serve with vegetables and/or cauliflower rice.

Bacon Cheese Chicken

Calories 302 – Protein 17g – Carbs 3g – Fat 24g

Servings: 10

Cooking: 6 hours

Ingredients:

- ¼ tsp. thyme
- ½ tsp. poultry seasoning
- ½ tsp. rosemary
- ¾ C. chicken broth
- 1 C. cheese
- 1 tsp. garlic
- 2-ounces cream cheese
- 2/3 C. heavy whipping cream
- 3 pieces of crumbled bacon
- 3 pieces of crumbled bacon
- 3 tbsp. butter
- 4-6 boneless skinless chicken breasts
- Pepper and salt

Preparation:

1. Place chicken into the bottom of your slowcooker along with butter, poultry seasonings, rosemary, thyme, garlic, and chicken broth.

2. Crumble 3 pieces of bacon onto the top of these components.

3. Set your pot to cook 6 hours on low.

4. When time is up, pour heavy whipping cream into the pot along with dollops of cream cheese. Stir to incorporate.

5. Shred chicken with forks within the slowcooker.

6. Grease a casserole dish.

7. Pour contents of your slowcooker into the greased dish.

8. Add a cup of cheddar cheese over the top along with another 3 pieces of crumbled bacon.

9. Put the dish in broiling over for 2-4 minutes to allow cheese to melt and become bubbly.

10. Top with extra bacon if you wish. Enjoy!

Chicken Peanut Curry

Calories 378 – Protein 21g – Carbs 6g – Fat 11g

Servings: 4

Cooking: 5 to 6 hours

Ingredients:

- ¼ C. cilantro
- ¼ tsp. red pepper flakes
- ½ C. red bell pepper
- ½ C. yellow onion
- ½ tsp. ginger
- ½ tsp. honey
- 1 14-ounce can coconut milk
- 1 C. snap peas
- 1 tbsp. basil leaves
- 1 tsp. curry powder
- 1 tsp. red Thai curry paste
- 2 tbsp. cashew, almond, or peanut butter
- 2 tbsp. tamari
- 4 pieces boneless skinless chicken breasts and thighs
- Lime juice
- Pepper and salt

Diet *Preparation:*

1. Mix honey, curry paste, curry powder, and coconut milk together.

2. Then add in tamari, nut butter of choice, ginger, and red pepper flakes to the mixture. Incorporate well and pour into slowcooker.

3. Chop up veggies and herbs.

4. Grate ginger.

5. Pour veggies, herbs, and ginger into your slowcooker.

6. Combine well.

7. Place in chicken breasts and thighs directly into the sauce. Immerse them in the sauce.

8. Cook 3 ½ - 4 hours on high or 5 ½ - 6 hours on low.

9. When time is up, stir all contents together. The chicken will fall apart.

10. Add in peas and let sit so they warm up before serving.

Keto Mexican Chicken

Calories 262 – Protein 32g – Carbs 8g – Fat 13g

Servings: 6

Cooking: 6 hours

Ingredients:

- ½ C. chicken stock
- 1 14-ounce can diced tomatoes with green chilies
- 1 C. sour cream
- 1 packet taco seasoning
- 2-pounds chicken breast

Preparation:

1. Set your slowcooker to low.

2. Pour in taco seasoning, tomatoes, chicken stock, and sour cream.

3. Stir well to combine.

4. Place chicken breasts into this mixture and spoon mixture over top of chicken breasts.

5. Cook for 6 hours on low.

Chicken Pad Thai with Vegetable Noodles

Calories 120 – Protein 19g – Carbs 2g – Fat 12g

Servings: 8

Cooking: 3 ½ - 4 hours

Ingredients:

- 1 bunch of green onion
- 1 C. chicken stock
- 1 C. coconut milk
- 1 carrot
- 1 handful bean sprouts
- 1 tbsp. coconut aminos
- 1 tsp. cayenne pepper
- 1 tsp. red pepper flakes
- 2 cloves garlic
- 2 tbsp. sunflower seed butter
- 2 tsp. fish sauce
- 2 tsp. powdered ginger
- 2 zucchinis
- 2-3 pounds chicken thighs or breasts

Preparation:

1. Season chicken with pepper and salt and a touch of cayenne pepper and ginger powder.

Add chicken stock and coconut milk to your slowcooker. Stir well.

2. Add green onion, red pepper, cayenne, garlic, ginger, fish sauce, coconut aminos, and sunflower seed butter. Stir well till butter dissolves.

3. Place chicken in the cooker.

4. Using a spiralizer, create noodles from zucchini. Shred carrots and wash bean sprouts.

5. Toss sprouts, carrots, and zucchini noodles together.

6. Balance vegetable noodles on top of the liquid in the pot. Press down just slightly. You want them steamed, not stewed.

7. Cook on low heat 3 ½ - 4 hours.

8. Remove chicken and chop into strips. Place chicken over noodles in a serving dish.

9. Garnish with cashews, cilantro and green onions if you desire.

Chicken and Sausage

Calories 456 – Protein 34g – Carbs 6g – Fat 18g

Servings: 5 to 6

Cooking: 4 to 6 hours

Ingredients:

- ½ C. white wine
- ½ tsp. salt
- 1 ½ pounds boneless, skinless chicken breasts
- 8-ounce package room-temp cream cheese
- 1 C. chicken stock
- 1 diced yellow onion
- 1 package andouille sausage
- 2 tbsp. grainy mustard
- 3 cloves minced garlic

Preparation:

1. Whip cream cheese with wine, mustard, salt, garlic and chicken stock.

2. Put chicken in the bottom of your slowcooker. Layer onions over the top.

3. Pour cream cheese mixture over onions and chicken.

4. Cook 5-6 hours on low or 4 hours on high.

Greek Chicken

Calories 321 – Protein 23g – Carbs 7g – Fat 12g

Servings: 4 to 5

Cooking: 6 hours

Ingredients:

- 1 ½ C. hot water
- 1 ½ tbsp. minced garlic
- 2 chicken bouillon cubes
- 3 tbsp. Greek rub
- 3 tbsp. lemon juice
- 3-4 boneless skinless chicken breasts

Preparation:

1. Grease your slowcooker.

2. Liberally rub breasts with Greek rub on all sides.

3. Place chicken in your slowcooker. Top with lemon juice.

4. Crumble bouillon cubes and mix with hot water. Make sure cubes dissolve and pour into pot.

5. Cook on low heat 6 hours.

6. When totally cooked, the chicken will be tenderized.

Garlic Butter Chicken in Cream Cheese Sauce

Calories 256 – Protein 19g – Carbs 6g – Fat 14g

Servings: 5

Cooking: 6 hours

Ingredients:

Chicken:

- 1 ½ tsp. salt
- 1 stick butter
- 2 – 2 ½ pounds of chicken breast
- 8 cloves garlic

Cream Cheese Sauce:

- 1 C. chicken stock
- 8 ounces cream cheese
- Salt

Preparation:

1. Put thawed chicken in the bottom of your slowcooker.

2. Put butter on top of chicken.

3. Put garlic into the pot, making sure to disperse evenly. Sprinkle with salt.

4. Cook on low heat 6 hours.

5. When time is up, take out chicken and place on a serving dish.

6. To make the sauce, mix stock with salt and cream cheese in a pan over intermediate warmth. Heat and stir until creamy.

7. Pour sauce over chicken and devour!

Chapter 9:
Beef Recipes

Slowcooker Keto Meatballs

Calories: 171 Carbs: 9g Fat: 17g Protein: 19g

Servings: 14

Cooking: 8 hours

Ingredients:

- ¼ C. mayo
- 1 egg
- 1-pound ground beef
- 1-pound ground pork
- 1 tsp. pepper
- 1 tsp. salt
- 14 grams crushed pork rinds
- 2 tbsp. grated parmesan cheese

Sauce:

- 12-ounce jar of sugar-free grape or raspberry jam
- 14-ounce jar chili sauce

Preparation:

1. Turn slowcooker on high. With olive oil, grease pot liberally.

2. Combine all recipe ingredients, minus sauce components, together well.

3. Roll mixture into 40-42 meatballs. Place meatballs in the slowcooker.

4. Mix together sauce ingredients until smooth and incorporated and pour over meatballs.

5. Set to cook on high 2-3 hours or set to cook on low 8 hours.

Keto Pot Roast

Calories: 307 Carbs: 1g Fat: 13g Protein: 10g

Servings: 4-5

Cooking: 4-5 hours

Ingredients:

- ½ C. mild pepper rings
- ½ C. beef broth
- ½ C. garlic butter
- ½ sliced onion
- 1 pack of ranch dressing mix
- 1 tbsp. olive oil
- 1-3 pounds of boneless beef roast

Preparation:

1. Pour oil in skillet and sear beef on all sides. Place into the slowcooker.

2. Pour other ingredients into the pot, stirring well to combine.

3. Cook 4-5 hours on high or 8-9 hours on low.

4. Shred with the help of two forks and devour!

Beef Short Ribs with Creamy Mushroom Sauce

Calories: 365 Carbs: 1g Fat: 33g Protein: 13g

Servings: 8

Cooking: 6-8 hours

Ingredients:

- ½ C. beef broth
- 1 tsp. garlic powder
- 1 tsp. pepper
- 1 tsp. salt
- 2 C. white mushrooms
- 2-pounds beef short ribs
- 3-ounces cream cheese

Preparation:

1. In a skillet, brown beef on all sides.

2. Mix together pepper, salt, garlic powder, mushrooms, broth, and cream cheese within your slowcooker.

3. Place ribs in the slowcooker.

4. Set to cook on low 6-8 hours. Ensure you mix things around every 1-2 hours during the cooking process.

Mushroom Pot Roast

Calories: 267 Carbs: 4g Fat: 16g Protein: 24g

Servings: 6

Cooking: 4 ½ - 5 hours

Ingredients:

- 1 tsp. onion powder
- 2 mushroom stock cubes + ½ C. water
- ¾ tsp salt
- 1 – 1 ½ pounds cremini mushrooms
- 1-2 tbsp. steak rub
- 2-3 tsp. olive oil
- 3 to 4- pound chuck roast
- ½ tsp. pepper

Preparation:

1. Pour mushroom cubes and water into a bowl. Pop in microwave and heat 60 seconds till dissolved. Stir well.

2. Trim fat from roast.

3. Mix up steak rub, pepper, salt, and onion powder together. Rub mixture onto roast.

4. Heat an iron skillet and brown meat on all sides for 5-7 minutes. Place meat into slowcooker.

5. Pour mushroom stock mixture into a pan, cooking 1-2 minutes. Scrape bits from bottom of the pan and pour over roast in the slowcooker.

6. Set to cook on high 3 hours.

7. Wash mushrooms and slice into thick pieces. Place over roast after 3 hours and cook another 45-60 minutes till mushrooms are cooked through, and the meat is nice and tender.

8. Scoop out meat with mushrooms. Strain juices.

9. Slice meat, place onto serving plates and top with cooked mushroom and a spoonful of cooking juices.

Beef and Broccoli

Calories: 564 Carbs: 6g Fat: 13g Protein: 26g

Servings: 3

Cooking: 2 hours

Ingredients:

- ¼ C. brown sugar
- ½ C. soy sauce
- 1 ½ pounds beef flank steak, thinly sliced
- 1 C. beef stock
- 2 tbsp. cornstarch
- 4 C. broccoli florets
- 5 minced garlic cloves

Preparation:

1. Add brown sugar, soy sauce, and beef stock to your slowcooker. Stir to combine. Then add beef and coat well with sauce.

2. Set to cook on high 2 hours.

3. Combine 2 tablespoons of cooking liquid with cornstarch.

4. Stir in cornstarch mixture along with garlic and broccoli.

5. Cook another half an hour till broccoli becomes tender.

Italian Beef

Calories 389 – Protein 39g – Carbs 7g – Fat 23g

Servings: 6 to 7

Cooking: 5-6 hours

Ingredients:

- ½ tsp. dried thyme
- 1 ½ C. crushed tomatoes
- 1 sliced white onion
- 1 tbsp. tomato paste
- 1 tsp. dried basil
- 1 tsp. dried oregano
- 1 tsp. garlic powder
- 1 tsp. salt
- 1/8 tsp. cinnamon
- 2 ½ - 3 pounds round beef roast
- 2 C. beef stock
- 2 C. chopped carrots
- 4-5 minced cloves garlic
- Pinch of red pepper flakes

Preparation:

1. Trim fat off roast. Cut into 3-4" chunks and add to slowcooker.

2. Mince garlic, chop and peel the carrots, and slice onion.

3. Add veggies to slowcooker.

4. Pour in all seasonings into the pot over top of veggies and meat.

5. Pour in tomatoes and stock. Add tomato paste and incorporate everything well.

6. Cook 5-6 hours on low. You should be able to easily shred meat when done.

Low Carb Beef Rags

Calories 289 – Protein 26g – Carbs 8g – Fat 11g

Serving: 6-8

Cooking: 4 hours

Ingredients:

- ½ tbsp. Dijon mustard
- ½ tbsp. pepper and salt
- 1 C. dry red wine
- 1 tsp. onion powder
- 2 tbsp. Worcestershire sauce
- 2 tsp. granulated garlic
- 3-pounds chuck arm pot roast
- 3 tbsp. extra-virgin olive oil

Preparation:

1. Use garlic, onion powder, pepper, and salt to season roast.

2. Ensure oven is preheated to 275 degrees.

3. Warm up 1 ½ tbsp. of oil in a Dutch oven.

   Sear roast for 3-4 minutes per side.

4. Add remaining olive oil halfway through searing meat.

5. Once meat is browned, put into your slowcooker. Then add in Dijon and drizzle with Worcestershire sauce.

6. Pour red wine over roast.

7. Cook on low heat 4-5 hours. Make sure to check your roast after 3 hours to see how tender it has become.

8. Once time is up, remove roast from pot. Using forks, pull roast into rags.

9. Discard bone and gristle but keep most of the fat. Stir meat into fat to incorporate.

10. Once you have shredded roast, stir in cooking juices.

Keto Beef Fajitas

Calories 257 – Protein 21g – Carbs 3g – Fat 10g

Servings: 6

Cooking: 8 hours

Ingredients:

- ½ C. onion
- 1 6-ounce can tomato paste
- 1 bouillon cube
- 1 tbsp. olive oil
- 1 tsp. oregano
- 1 tsp. salt
- 2 green peppers
- 2 red peppers
- 3-pounds beef stew or cubed chuck roast
- 4 cloves garlic
- Pepper

Preparation:

1. Pour all recipe components into your slowcooker.

   Set cooking heat to low.

2. Cook 8 hours till meat begins to fall apart and is very tender.

3. Season with pepper and salt to achieve the desired flavor.

4. Serve simply in a bowl or on tortillas with avocado and sour cream.

Spicy Swiss Steak

Calories 348 – Protein 24g – Carbs 8g – Fat 17g

Servings: 6

Cooking: 8 hours

Ingredients:

- ½ C. bell pepper
- ½ C. carrots
- ½ C. celery
- ½ C. onion
- ½ tsp. salt
- 1 1/3 C. beef broth
- 1 14.5-ounce can Rotel tomatoes
- 1 tbsp. liquid smoke in mesquite flavor
- 2 ½-pounds boneless round steak
- 2 minced cloves garlic
- Several pinches of pepper

Preparation:

1. Pour in all components directly into your slowcooker

2. Stir gently to incorporate.

3. Set cooker to low and cook 8-10 hours.

4. When time is up, take out and shred with forks or eat whole.

Barbacoa Beef

Calories 298 – Protein 24g – Carbs 6g – Fat 11g

Servings: 6

Cooking: 4 hours

Ingredients:

- ½ C. water
- ½ tbsp. cumin
- ½ tsp. cloves
- ½ tsp. pepper
- 1 can chipotle chilies in adobo sauce
- 1 tsp. salt
- 2 ½ - 3-pounds boneless chuck roast
- 2 tbsp. lime juice
- 2 tbsp. olive oil
- 2 tsp. oregano
- 3 tbsp. tomato paste
- 4 garlic cloves

Preparation:

1. Blend together all above components minus chicken in a blender.

2. Put roast into your slow cooker. Add sauce all around the meat, ensuring a good covering.

3. Set slowcooker on high to cook 4 hours. The roast will begin to pull apart and become tenderized.

4. Shred meat in a bowl and pour sauce over the top. Season with pinches of pepper and salt till you achieve desired taste.

Bison Meatloaf

Calories 137 – Protein 13g – Carbs 1g – Fat 9g

Servings: 6-8

Cooking: 3 hours

Ingredients:

- ½ C. fresh parsley
- ½ C. parmesan cheese
- ½ tsp. pepper and salt
- 1 C. zucchini
- 1 tbsp. dried oregano
- 2 eggs
- 2-pounds lean ground sirloin or bison
- 2 tbsp. onion powder
- 3 tbsp. balsamic vinegar
- 4 cloves garlic
- Olive oil

Topping:

- ¼ C. shredded mozzarella cheese
- ¼ C. tomato sauce or ketchup
- 2 tbsp. parsley

Preparation:

1. Line bottom of your slowcooker with strips of foil. Generously spray foil with non-stick cooking spray.

2. Combine all recipe components minus toppings ingredients. The mixture will be wet and loose.

3. Pour mixture into your slowcooker and with your hands form a meatloaf shape. Cover pot.

4. Cook 3 hours on high or 6 hours on low.

5. At 15 minutes on the timer, shut off the pot and take off the lid.

6. Pour ketchup and cheese over top of the meatloaf.

7. Let sit 10-15 minutes till cheese melts.

8. Take out meatloaf and cut into slices.

9. Garnish with parsley.

Chapter 10: Pork Recipes

Cuban Mojo Pork

Calories: 294 Carbs: 7g Fat: 37g Protein: 51g

Servings: 8

Cooking: 6 ½ - 7 hours

Ingredients:

- ¼ C. chopped cilantro
- ½ C. lime juice
- ½ C. olive oil
- ¾ C. orange juice
- 1 ½ tsp. salt
- 1 bone-in pork shoulder
- 1 tsp. pepper
- 2 tsp. cumin
- 2 tsp. oregano
- 8 finely cloves of garlic
- Zest of 1 lime
- Zest of 1 orange

Preparation:

1. Make a few slits into the pork with a knife.

2. Add all other components to slowcooker. Mix well to incorporate.

3. Gently place pork among ingredients in the pot. With a spoon, ladle liquids over pork.

4. Cook 5-6 hours on high or 8-10 hours on low.

5. Remove pork from slowcooker and place on a sheet lined with foil.

6. Bake at 400 degrees 15-20 minutes till browned.

7. Allow to rest 10-15 minutes before serving!

Pork Chili Verde

Calories: 278 Carbs: 3g Fat: 25g Protein: 19g

Servings: 4-6

Cooking: 6 ½ - 7 hours

Ingredients:

- ½ C. broth
- ¾ C. diced onion
- 1 pound chopped tomatillos
- 1 tbsp. olive oil
- 2 minced Serrano peppers
- 2 pounds pork stew meat
- 2-3 tbsp. cilantro
- 3 minced cloves garlic

Preparation:

1. Warm up slowcooker and add all recipe components into pot minus the cilantro and broth. Sauté 5 minutes. Then add cilantro and broth.

2. Close lid and set to cook 6 to 7 hours on low heat till tender and well combined.

3. Stir well and serve warm with cheese, salsa, and avocado!

Korean Spicy Pork

Calories: 189 Carbs: 7g Fat: 9g Protein: 15g

Servings: 4

Cooking: 2-3 hours

Ingredients:

Marinating and Cooking:

- 2 tbsp. gochujang
- 2 packets Splenda
- 1 tbsp. sesame oil
- 1 tbsp. rice wine
- 1 tbsp. soy sauce
- 1 tbsp. minced garlic
- 1 tbsp. minced ginger
- 1 thinly sliced onion
- 1-pound pork shoulder, sliced into cubes
- ¼ C. water
- ¼ - 1 tsp. cayenne pepper

Finishing:

- ¼ C. sliced green onions
- 1 tbsp. sesame seeds
- 1 thinly sliced onion

Preparation:

1. Mix up all marinade and cooking components in your slowcooker. Let mixture sit 60 minutes.

2. Set to cook on high 2-3 hours.

3. Warm up a cast iron skillet. Add pork cubes to skillet along with the onion. Pour in ¼ - ½ cup of sauce.

4. Once the sauce has reduced, and onions are soft, sprinkle sesame seeds and green onions.

Pulled Pork Sliders

Calories 257 – Protein 21g – Carbs 6g – Fat 24g

Servings: 8

Cooking: 8 hours

Ingredients:

Pulled Pork:

- ½ tsp. cayenne
- 1 onion
- 1 tsp. paprika
- 1 tsp. pepper
- 2 tsp. chili powder
- 2 tsp. cumin
- 2 tsp. oregano
- 2 tsp. salt
- 3 minced cloves garlic
- Juice of 1 lemon
- Juice of 1 lime
- Large pork roast

Buns:

- ¼ tsp. cumin
- ¼ tsp. paprika
- 1 good-sized sweet potato

- 2 tbsp. coconut oil

Preparation:

1. To make pork, mix all spices together and then rub onto roast.

2. Layer onions in the bottom of slowcooker.

3. Squeeze half of the citrus juices over onions.

4. Place roast in the slowcooker over onions and then squeeze remaining citrus juices over meat.

5. Cook 8 hours on low.

6. When time is up, shred meat with forks.

7. To make buns, slice up the sweet potato into ¼" pieces.

8. With parchment paper, line a tray.

9. Bake at 350 degrees for 10 minutes till just crispy.

10. Place a helping of roast on buns and devour!

Shredded Taco Pork

Calories 190 – Protein 18g – Carbs 4g – Fat 11g

Servings: 10

Cooking: 9 hours

Ingredients:

- ¼ C. grass-fed butter
- 1 packet taco seasoning
- 2 C. chicken stock
- 4-pounds pork roast

Preparation:

1. Turn on your slowcooker to low.

2. Place pork roast in your slowcooker.

3. Top with taco seasoning, butter, and chicken stock.

4. Cover and cook 8-10 hours.

5. One time is up, remove and shred pork. Utilize for a variety of meals!

Pork Adobado

Calories 243 – Protein 33g – Carbs 6g – Fat 10g

Servings: 8

Cooking: 8 hours

Ingredients:

- ¼ C. cilantro
- 1 onion
- 1 tbsp. coriander
- 1 tsp. cumin
- 1 tsp. dried oregano
- 2 bay leaves
- 2 chipotle peppers
- 2 dried ancho chile peppers
- 3 pounds lean pork shoulder
- 6 garlic cloves

Preparation:

1. Toast chilies for 3-5 minutes in a pan till fragrant. Allow to cool and remove seeds and stem.

2. Add chilies to a pot and cover with water. Heat up to the boiling point let simmer for 5 minutes.

3. Take chilies away from heat and let rest in water for half an hour.

4. Add onion, oregano, garlic, coriander, cumin, chipotles, 1 cup of reserved cooking liquid and chili peppers to a blender, combining well. Blend to combine. You have now created adobo sauce!

5. Season pork with pepper and salt. Pour a bit of adobo sauce into the bottom of the pot, adding pork shoulder over the top of sauce and pouring remaining sauce over meat.

6. Cook on low for 6 to 8 hours till pork is tender.

7. When the timer goes off, use forks to pull pork apart. Mix with sauce.

Dry Rub Baby Back Ribs

Calories 243 – Protein 41g – Carbs 8g – Fat 37g

Servings: 2

Cooking: 2 hours

Ingredients:

- 1 rack of baby back ribs
- 1 tbsp. chili powder
- 1 tbsp. paprika
- 1 tsp. cayenne pepper
- 1 tsp. garlic
- 1 tsp. ground mustard
- 1 tsp. pepper
- 1 tsp. Splenda brown sugar blend
- 2 tbsp. cumin

Preparation:

1. Combine all spices. Rub onto the rack of ribs, coating thoroughly.

2. Wrap ribs in foil and pop in fridge 4 hours or overnight.

3. Ensure slowcooker is set to high heat.

4. Unwrap ribs and set into the bottom of slowcooker.

5. Cook 2 hours on high until meat begins to fall off the bone.

6. If the meat is not quite done, cook in 15-minute intervals till you reach the desired doneness. Devour! (And don't skimp on the napkins!)

Jamaican Jerk Pork

Calories 282 – Protein 23g – Carbs 8g – Fat 20g

Servings: 12

Cooking: 2 hours

Ingredients:

- ¼ C. Jamaican Jerk spice blend
- ½ C. beef broth
- 1 tbsp. olive oil
- 4-pound pork shoulder

Preparation:

1. Rub spice blend and olive oil over pork shoulder.

2. In a pan, sear shoulder on all sides.

3. Add beef broth to your pot and place pork into the broth.

4. Cover and cook 2 hours till meat is tender and falls right off the bone.

5. Shred with forks and eat!

Pulled Pork Carnitas

Calories 256 – Protein 32g – Carbs 11g – Fat 21g

Servings: 8

Cooking: 3 hours

Ingredients:

- 1 C. chicken broth
- 2 tbsp. grapeseed oil
- 5-pound pork shoulder

Seasoning Salt:

- 1 tbsp. garlic powder
- 1 tbsp. pepper
- 3 tbsp. salt

Preparation:

1. Mix seasoning salt ingredients together. Rub onto pork.

2. Turn on the slowcooker, adding oil and warming until sizzling. Place pork in the cooker and sauté 3-5 minutes. Flip and pour broth into the pot.

3. Cover and cook about 3 hours till pork is tender.

4. Remove pork and let rest half an hour. Shred and devour!

Smothered Pork Chops

Calories 302 – Protein 30g – Carbs 10g – Fat 24g

Servings: 6

Cooking: 4 hours

Ingredients:

- ¼ C. butter
- ½ C. buttermilk
- 1-3 tbsp. almond flour
- 1-pound pork chops
- 2 C. chicken stock
- 2-3 C. chopped veggies of choice (mushrooms, peppers, onions, etc.)
- Olive oil
- Seasoned almond flour

Preparation:

1. In seasoned flour, dredge pork chops.

2. Heat up oil in slowcooker. Sear chops till browned and set to the side.

3. Pour in more oil into the pot and sauté veggies until caramelized. Sprinkle almond flour over vegetables, stirring constantly 60 seconds. Then pour the stock into the slowcooker.

4. Season stock with pepper, salt, and buttermilk.

5. Cook mixture 4 hours.

6. Place on serving plates topped with cooking juices.

Juicy Pork Tenderloin

Calories 256 – Protein 29g – Carbs 8g – Fat 18g

Servings: 4-6

Cooking: 3 ½ - 4 hours

Ingredients:

- 1 ½ pounds pork tenderloin
- 1 ½ tsp. chia seeds
- 1 C. chicken broth
- 1 minced garlic clove
- 1 tbsp. seasoning blend of choice
- 1 tbsp. Worcestershire sauce
- 2 tbsp. Dijon mustard
- 2 tbsp. sugar-free honey
- 3 tbsp. water

Preparation:

1. Trim pork. Mix Worcestershire sauce, sugar-free honey, mustard, chicken broth, seasoning blend, and garlic together.

2. Place tenderloin into slowcooker and coat with sugar-free honey sauce.

3. Close pot and cook 3 to 4 hours on high heat.

4. If you want shredded pork, remove 6-8 minutes before cooking time is up. Take out tenderloin.

5. Mix water and chia seeds together. Whisk into cooking juices in the slowcooker, cooking 1-2 minutes till it turns into gravy.

6. Slice pork tenderloin and spoon gravy onto meat.

Buttery Ranch Boneless Pork Chops

Calories 216 – Protein 23g – Carbs 6g – Fat 24g

Servings: 5

Cooking: 4-5 hours

Ingredients:

- 1 C. water
- 1 package ranch mix
- 1 stick butter
- 1 tbsp. coconut oil
- 4-6 boneless pork chops

Preparation:

1. Put pork chops into the slowcooker along with coconut oil. Heat cooker and brown sides.

2. Put butter over chops and sprinkle with ranch mix. Pour water over pork.

3. Set to cook on high 4 to 5 hours until tender.

4. Spoon butter sauce over pork chops when serving.

Chapter 11:
Seafood Recipes

Creamy Tomato Seafood Bisque

Calories: 345 Carbs: 3g Fat: 15g Protein: 10g

Servings: 3-4

Cooking: 45 minutes – 1 hour

Ingredients:

- 1 bay leaf
- 1 chopped onion
- 1 minced garlic clove
- 1 peeled and chopped carrot
- 2 chopped celery stalks
- 2 tbsp. flour
- 2 tsp. oregano
- 2 tsp. sherry
- 29-ounce can diced tomatoes
- 3-pounds seafood of choice (I like using bay scallops and shrimp)
- 5 tbsp. butter
- 6 C. chicken broth
- 8-ounces cream cheese

Preparation:

1. Add butter, veggies and bay leaf to slowcooker. Cook on high half an hour.

2. Add flour, stir for a few minutes and add broth, oregano, and tomatoes. Cook another half an hour.

3. Add cream cheese and sherry, allowing cheese to melt. Cook 10 minutes.

4. Discard bay leaf. With an immersion blender, puree mixture until smooth.

5. Add scallops and shrimp. Cook 20-30 minutes to heat through.

6. Garnish with parsley and season with pepper and salt before serving.

Seafood Cioppino

Calories: 167 Carbs: 1g Fat: 19g Protein: 12g

Servings: 3-4

Cooking: 7 hours

Ingredients:

- ½ C. chopped parsley
- ½ C. dry white wine
- ½ tsp. salt
- 1 diced yellow onion
- 1-pound haddock fillets
- 1-pound raw shrimp
- 2 6.5-ounce cans minced clams in clam juice
- 2 bay leaves
- 2 chopped celery stalks
- 2 tbsp. olive oil
- 2 tsp. Italian seasoning
- 2 tsp. red wine vinegar
- 28-ounce can diced tomatoes
- 3 tbsp. tomato paste
- 6 minced garlic cloves
- 8-ounces clam juice
- 8-ounces lump crab meat

Preparation:

1. Mix salt, bay leaves, Italian seasoning, olive oil, vinegar, garlic, white wine, tomato paste, clam juice, celery, onions, and tomatoes in the slowcooker.

2. Set to cook on low 6 hours.

3. Mix in crab meat, clams, shrimp, and haddock. Cook another 45 minutes till shrimp is pink and haddock flakes with a fork easily.

4. Discard bay leaves and spoon into serving bowls.

Tilapia with Roasted Pepper Sauce

Calories: 251 Carbs: 2g Fat: 18g Protein: 11g

Servings: 3-4

Cooking: 1 ½ hours

Ingredients:

- ½ C. grated parmesan cheese
- ¾ C. heavy cream
- 1 diced onion
- 1-pound tilapia fillets
- 2 chopped garlic cloves
- 3 tbsp. butter
- 6-ounces chopped roasted peppers
- 6-ounces pureed roasted peppers

Preparation:

1. Add 2 tablespoons butter to skillet. Warm up and add tilapia fillets, cooking 3-4 minutes per side till thoroughly cooked.

2. Season fillets with pepper and salt. Set to the side.

3. To the same skillet, add remaining butter along with the onion. Sauté 5 minutes.

4. Add garlic to onion along with pureed and chopped roasted peppers, cooking 5 minutes.

5. Pour in parmesan cheese and heavy cream. Turn off heat, stir, and adjust seasoning if needed.

6. Add everything to slowcooker and cook on high 1 hour.

7. Garnish with parsley and more parmesan cheese.

Lemon Pepper Salmon

Calories: 165 Carbs: 1g Fat: 8g Protein: 13g

Servings: 3-4

Cooking: 1-2 hours

Ingredients:

- ¼ tsp. salt
- ½ thinly sliced lemon
- ½ tsp. pepper
- ¾ C. water
- 1 carrot
- 1 red bell pepper
- 1 zucchini
- 1-pound salmon skin-on fillet
- 3 tsp. ghee
- Few springs of basil, tarragon, dill, and parsley

Preparation:

1. Place water and herbs into the slowcooker. Place salmon over herbs, skin side down.

2. Drizzle fillet with ghee and season with pepper and salt. Cover with lemon slices.

3. Set to cook on high 1-2 hours.

4. While salmon cooks, julienne cut your veggies.

5. Add veggies to slowcooker and cook another hour on high.

6. Serve salmon with lemon slices and sliced veggies.

Garlic Shrimp

Calories: 277 Carbs: 2g Fat: 9g Protein: 14g

Servings: 6-8

Cooking: 30 minutes

Ingredients:

- ¼ tsp. pepper
- ¼ tsp. crushed red pepper flakes
- ¾ C. extra-virgin olive oil
- 1 tbsp. parsley
- 1 tsp. salt
- 1 tsp. smoked paprika
- 2-pounds peeled and deveined large shrimp
- 6 thinly sliced garlic cloves

Preparation:

1. Mix red pepper flakes, pepper, salt, paprika, garlic, and oil together within slowcooker. Set to cook on high for half an hour.

2. Mix in shrimp, mixing well.

3. Cook 10 minutes on high. Cooking another 10 minutes, stirring until shrimp turn opaque.

4. Place in a serving bowl, pour some sauce over and garnish with parsley.

Shrimp Fajitas

Calories: 308 Carbs: 5g Fat: 18g Protein: 27g

Servings: 4

Cooking: 5- 6 ½ hours

Ingredients:

- ½ C. chicken broth
- ½ tsp. paprika
- 1 packet taco seasoning
- 1-pound deveined and peeled raw shrimp
- 1 quartered tomato
- 1 sliced onion
- 1 tsp. chili powder
- 1 tsp. salt
- 2 sliced green peppers
- 2 sliced red peppers

Preparation:

1. Pour all ingredients minus shrimp into your Slowcooker. Set to cook on low 5-6 hours.

2. Add shrimp, mixing gently.

3. Cook on high 30-45 more minutes.

Clam Chowder

Calories: 226 Carbs: 6g Fat: 18g Protein: 21g

Servings: 4

Cooking: 1 ½ hours

Ingredients:

- 1 ½ C. diced onion
- 1-quart chicken broth
- 1 tbsp. salt
- 1 tbsp. whole, dried thyme
- 16-ounces bottled clam juice
- 2-pounds frozen cauliflower florets
- 3 cans whole clams
- 4 garlic cloves
- 4-5 C. peeled and diced celeriac root
- 8-ounces chopped bacon
- Pinch of cayenne pepper

Preparation:

1. Dice up onions and peel and dice celeriac root into ¼-inch pieces/

2. Sauté bacon in pan 5-7 minutes till crispy. Place on paper towel to drain.

3. Pour cauliflower florets and broth into your slowcooker.

4. Set to cook on high 1 hour. Remove and pour into a blender along with garlic. Blend until smooth and set to the side.

5. Add onion and celeriac root to slowcooker. Then add cayenne pepper, clam juice, pepper, thyme, and salt. Mix well. Set to cook on high 1 hour.

6. Add cooked bacon and cauliflower puree. Stir everything well to incorporate thoroughly.

7. Pour clams into a sieve and rinse well. Roughly chop clams and mix into chowder.

8. Adjust seasonings to satisfy your taste buds.

Coconut Milk Shrimp

Calories: 192 Carbs: 4g Fat: 12g Protein: 16g

Servings: 4

Cooking: 3-4 hours

Ingredients:

- ½ can unsweetened coconut milk
- ½ tsp. cayenne pepper
- ½ tsp. turmeric
- 1-pound deveined and shelled shrimp
- 1 tbsp. minced garlic
- 1 tbsp. minced ginger
- 1 tsp. garam masala
- 1 tsp. salt

Preparation:

1. Mix all ingredients together till well combined.

2. Pour contents into your slowcooker.

3. Cook 7 hours on low or 3 ½ - 4 hours on high.

Orange Ginger Salmon

Calories: 166 Carbs: 0g Fat: 8g Protein: 23g

Servings: 4

Cooking: 2 ½ hours

Ingredients:

- ½ - 1 tsp. salt
- 1 – 1 ½ tsp. pepper
- 1-pound salmon
- 1 tbsp. soy sauce
- 1 tsp. minced garlic
- 2 tbsp. low-sugar marmalade
- 2 tsp. minced ginger

Preparation:

1. Place salmon into a Ziploc baggie.

2. Mix up all other ingredients and pour into bag with salmon. Marinate 20-30 minutes.

3. Place salmon along with marinade sauce into your slowcooker.

4. Set to cook on low 2 hours.

5. Ensure oven is preheated to broil.

6. Place salmon into a piece of foil and broil 3-4 minutes to crisp.

Seafood Gumbo

Calories: 343 Carbs: 9g Fat: 12g Protein: 49g

Servings: 8

Cooking: 7 hours

Ingredients:

- ¼ C. tomato paste
- 1 ½ C. bone broth
- 2 diced bell peppers
- 2 diced yellow onions
- 2-pounds deveined raw shrimp
- 24-ounces sea bass fillets, cut into 2-inch chunks
- 28-ounces diced tomatoes
- 3 bay leaves
- 3 tbsp. Cajun seasoning
- 3 tbsp. ghee
- 4 diced celery ribs

Preparation:

1. Season fillets with pepper and salt, sprinkling half of Cajun seasoning.

2. Place ghee into the skillet and sauté fillet chunks 4 minutes. Add remaining Cajun seasoning with celery, pepper, and onions, sautéing 2 minutes till fragrant.

3. Add broth, bay leaves, tomato paste, diced tomatoes, and cooked fish to slowcooker. Then mix in all remaining ingredients, stirring to incorporate.

4. Set to cook on low 7 hours.

Chapter 12: Side Dish Recipes

Parmesan Zucchini Tots

Calories: 175 Carbs: 1g Fat: 19g Protein: 11g

Servings: 10

Cooking: 3-4 hours

Ingredients:

- ½ C. shredded parmesan cheese
- ½ tbsp. Italian seasoning
- 1 ½ C. shredded zucchini
- 1 C. panko breadcrumbs
- 1 egg

Preparation:

1. Add shredded zucchini to slowcooker.

2. Combine with remaining ingredients, mixing thoroughly.

3. Set to cook on high 3-4 hours till zucchini is tender.

4. Remove mixture and shape into small "tot" shapes.

5. Line a sheet with parchment paper and bake 15-20 minutes at 400 degrees till crispy.

Bacon Gouda Cauliflower Mash

Calories: 147 Carbs: 2g Fat: 10g Protein: 7g

Servings: 4-6

Cooking: 4 hours

Ingredients:

- ¼ tsp. garlic powder
- ¼ tsp. pepper
- ½ tsp. salt
- 1/3 C. shredded smoked gouda cheese
- 2 tbsp. butter
- 3 tbsp. heavy cream
- 4 C. cauliflower florets
- 4 slices cooked bacon

Preparation:

1. Place everything into your slowcooker and mix thoroughly.

2. Cook 4 hours on high.

3. With a potato masher, gently mash mixture till just slightly chunky.

Cauliflower Hummus

Calories: 97 Carbs: 0g Fat: 12g Protein: 5g

Servings: 10

Cooking: 4 hours

Ingredients:

- ½ tsp. salt
- ¾ tsp. salt
- 1 ½ tbsp. tahini paste
- 2 crushed garlic cloves
- 2 tbsp. avocado oil
- 2 tbsp. water
- 3 C. cauliflower florets
- 3 garlic cloves
- 3 tbsp. extra-virgin olive oil
- 3 tbsp. lemon juice

Preparation:

1. Place all recipe components into your slowcooker.

2. Cook 4 hours on high.

3. With an immersion blender, blend mixture until creamy and smooth.

Coconut Lime Cauliflower Rice

Calories: 215 Carbs: 2g Fat: 14g Protein: 8g

Servings: 9

Cooking: 4-5 hours

Ingredients:

- 1 tbsp. chopped cilantro
- 2 C. chopped cauliflower
- 2 tbsp. coconut oil
- 2 tbsp. water
- 2 tsp. lime zest
- 3 tbsp. coconut milk powder

Preparation:

1. Combine all ingredients in your slowcooker.

2. Set to cook on high 4-5 hours.

Celery Cauliflower Puree

Calories: 167 Carbs: 1g Fat: 8g Protein: 4g

Servings: 6-8

Cooking: 5 hours

Ingredients:

- ½ tsp. salt
- 1 celery root sliced into ½-inch cubes
- 1 head cauliflower sliced into florets
- 3 tbsp. butter

Preparation:

1. Add all ingredients to slowcooker and combine.

2. Set to cook on high 5 hours till cauliflower and celery root is tender.

3. With an immersion blender, slightly blend mixture until smooth.

Parmesan and Chive Mashed Cauliflower

Calories: 190 Carbs: 2g Fat: 18g Protein: 7g

Servings: 4-6

Cooking: 2-3 hours

Ingredients:

- ¼ C. chopped chives
- ¼ C. grated parmesan cheese
- 2 C. chicken broth
- 2 small cauliflower heads, cored and sliced into florets

Preparation:

1. Add all ingredients to slowcooker, stir well.

2. Set to cook on high 2-3 hours.

3. Season with pepper and salt and sprinkle with additional parmesan.

Pepper Jack Cauliflower

Calories: 272 Carbs: 6g Fat: 21g Protein: 11g

Servings: 6

Cooking: 1 hour

Ingredients:

- ¼ C. whipping cream
- ½ tsp. pepper
- 1 head cauliflower, sliced into 1-inch florets
- 1 tsp. salt
- 2 tbsp. butter
- 4 -ounces cream cheese
- 4-ounces shredded pepper jack cheese
- 6 slices cooked and crumbled bacon

Preparation:

1. Grease your slowcooker.

2. Add all ingredients except pepper jack cheese to slowcooker. Stir well.

3. Set to cook on low 3 hours.

4. Stir in pepper jack cheese and cook another 30-60 minutes until cauliflower is nice and tender.

5. Stir in bacon crumbles and serve.

Keto Stuffing

Calories: 256 Carbs: 2g Fat: 21g Protein: 9g

Servings: 10

Cooking: 3-4 hours

Ingredients:

- 2 eggs
- Fresh herbs of choice
- ¼ C. parsley
- 12 C. cubed tempeh
- 2 C. chopped celery
- 2 diced onions
- 2 tsp. poultry seasoning
- 1 C. butter
- 3-4 C. chicken broth
- ½ tsp. salt
- ½ tsp. pepper

Preparation:

1. Heat butter in a pan and add pepper, salt, and poultry seasoning. Stir well. Add onions and celery to pan, sautéing till soft. Allow to cool completely.

2. In a bowl, add tempeh cubes with cooled celery and onions. Mix in parsley and chicken broth. Then add in eggs.

3. Cover and chill overnight for tempeh to marinate.

4. Grease your slowcooker well. Add stuffing mixture to the pot.

5. Set to cook on low 3-4 hours.

Keto Green Beans

Calories: 101 Carbs: 1g Fat: 11g Protein: 4g

Servings: 6

Cooking: 4-5 hours

Ingredients"

- 1 diced yellow onion
- 1 tbsp. butter
- 14.4-ounce can chicken broth
- 2 minced garlic cloves
- 2-pounds fresh green beans

Preparation:

1. Sauté garlic and onion together 7-10 minutes. Add to slowcooker.

2. Add green beans and chicken broth to slowcooker.

3. Set to cook on low 4-5 hours. Season as needed.

Cheesy Bacon Cauliflower

Calories: 278 Carbs: 2g Fat: 17g Protein: 6g

Servings: 6

Cooking: 3-4 hour

Ingredients:

- ¼ C. all-purpose flour
- ¼ C. butter
- ¼ tsp. pepper
- ½ tsp. salt
- 1 ½ C. grated mozzarella cheese
- 2 C. milk
- 2-pounds cauliflower florets
- 3-ounces bacon crumbles

Preparation:

1. Place cauliflower florets in the slowcooker.

2. In a pan, melt butter and mix in pepper, salt, and flour. Add milk and simmer until mixture begins to bubble. Add cheese and stir until smooth. Pour over cauliflower and combine.

3. Set to cook on low 3-4 hours.

4. Mix in bacon. Season as desired.

Chapter 13:
Sweet Recipes

Lemon Cheesecake Mousse

Calories: 156 Carbs: 1g Fat: 17g Protein: 14g

Servings: 5-7

Cooking: 30 minutes

Ingredients:

- ¼ C. lemon juice
- ½ - 1 tsp lemon liquid stevia
- 1 C. heavy cream
- 1/8 tsp. salt
- 8-ounces cream cheese

Preparation:

1. To a mixer, add lemon juice and cream cheese. Blend until smooth. Add heavy cream along with remaining components, blending till well incorporated.

2. Adjust sweetener if needed.

3. Pour into slowcooker. Set to cook on low 30 minutes.

4. Pour into serving glasses and chill 5 hours or overnight.

5. Serve topped with lemon zest.

Keto-fied Apple Cider

Calories: 178 Carbs: 1g Fat: 8g Protein: 5g

Servings: 12-15

Cooking: 3 hours

Ingredients:

- ¼ C. coconut sugar
- ¼ C. maple syrup
- 1 sliced naval orange
- 1 tsp. allspice berries
- 2 tsp. whole cloves
- 3 cinnamon sticks
- 6 apples of choice, cored and sliced
- 7 C. water

Preparation:

1. Pour all ingredients into your slowcooker and pour water over everything.

2. Set to cook on high 3 hours.

3. Discard orange slices and cinnamon sticks.

4. With an immersion blender, blend mixture until smooth.

5. Cook for another hour on high.

6. Strain mixture through cheesecloth.

7. Add back to the pot to keep warm.

Chocolate Chip Blueberry Cake

Calories: 289 Carbs: 5g Fat: 19g Protein: 9g

Servings: 10-12

Cooking: 3 hours

Ingredients:

- ¼ C. chocolate whey protein powder
- ¼ C. melted butter
- ¼ C. melted coconut oil
- ¼ tsp. salt
- ½ C. heavy cream
- ½ swerve sweetener
- 1 C. blackberries
- 1 C. unsweetened shredded coconut
- 1/3 C. dark chocolate chips (sugar-free)
- 2 C. almond flour
- 2 tsp. baking soda
- 4 eggs

Preparation:

1. Grease inside of slowcooker with butter.

2. Mix all of the dry ingredients together. Then add in all wet components, blending well to ensure adequate incorporation.

3. Pour batter into prepared slowcooker.

4. Set to cook on low 3 hours.

5. Top with additional blueberries before indulging.

Zesty Lemon Cake

Calories: 250 Carbs: 2g Fat: 16g Protein: 11g

Servings: 10

Cooking: 6-8 hours

Ingredients:

- ¼ C. coconut flour
- ¼ C. plain egg protein powder
- ½ C. unsweetened almond milk
- ½ C. swerve sweetener
- 1 tsp. baking soda
- 1/3 C. butter
- 2 C. almond flour
- 2 tsp. cream of tartar
- 2 tsp. vanilla extract
- 4 eggs
- Zest of 1 lemon

Filling:

- 1 C. coconut cream
- 1 C. low-carb lemon curd
- 1 tsp. vanilla extract

Glaze:

- ½ C. coconut butter
- 1 tbsp. lemon juice
- 2 tbsp. coconut oil
- 2 tbsp. swerve sweetener
- Zest of 1 lemon

Preparation:

1. Combine almond milk and butter together. Then mix in vanilla, eggs, and lemon zest.

2. Combine all dry components together. Then combine wet and dry mixtures, combining well.

3. Line a springform pan with parchment paper and pour batter into it.

4. Place pan into the slowcooker and cook on low 2 hours.

5. Take out and place in fridge 4-6 hour to chill.

6. To prepare filling, combine all ingredients together until smooth. Do the same with glaze.

7. Cut cake in half. Fill one part of the cake with filling, lay the other half over the top and then drizzle with glaze. Tip with additional lemon zest.

Keto Slowcooker Cheesecake

Calories: 301 Carbs: 2g Fat: 31g Protein: 23g

Servings: 12

Cooking: 2-3 hours

Ingredients:

- ½ tbsp. vanilla extract
- 1 C. Splenda
- 3 8-ounce packages of cream cheese
- 3 eggs

Preparation:

1. Allow cream cheese to warm up to room temperature.

2. Mix sugar and cream cheese together until well blended. Mix in one egg at a time, making sure to beat well after every addition.

3. Add vanilla and mix well.

4. Grease a pan or bowl well and add cream cheese mixture to it.

5. Add 2-3 cups of water into the bottom of slowcooker.

6. Add pan to pot. Set to cook on high 2 – 2 ½ hours.

Creamy Pumpkin Custard

Calories: 419 Carbs: 4g Fat: 16g Protein: 19g

Servings: 8-10

Cooking: 2-3 hours

Ingredients:

- 4 tbsp. butter
- 1 tsp. pumpkin pie spice
- ½ C. almond flour
- 1 tsp. vanilla extract
- 1 C. pumpkin puree
- ½ C. granulated stevia
- 4 eggs
- 1/8 tsp. salt

Preparation:

1. Grease inside of slowcooker.

2. Beat eggs until smooth. Then beat in sweetener gradually. Add vanilla and pumpkin puree until blended well.

3. Then mix in pumpkin pie spice, salt, and almond flour. Blend as you add in butter. Pour into slowcooker.

4. Place a paper towel over the opening of the pot before closing it.

5. Cook 2-3 hours on low.

6. Serve warm with whipped cream and a dash of nutmeg!

Chocolate Molten Lava Cake

Calories: 418 Carbs: 4g Fat: 27g Protein: 8g

Servings: 12

Cooking: 3 hours

Ingredients:

- ½ C. melted and cooled butter
- ½ C. flour
- ½ tsp. salt
- ½ tsp. vanilla liquid stevia
- 1 ½ C. swerve sweetener
- 1 tsp. baking powder
- 1 tsp. vanilla extract
- 2 C. hot water
- 3 egg yolks
- 3 whole eggs
- 4-ounces sugar-free chocolate chips
- 5 tbsp. unsweetened cocoa powder

Preparation:

1. Grease slowcooker liberally.

2. Whisk baking powder, salt, 3 tbsp. cocoa powder, flour, and 1 ¼ C. swerve together.

3. Stir liquid stevia, vanilla, yolks, eggs, and melted butter together.

4. Combine wet and dry mixture till well incorporated. Pour into slowcooker.

5. Top with chocolate chips. Mix in the remaining swerve and cocoa powder.

6. Set to cook on low 3 hours.

Lemon Slowcooker Cake

Calories: 310 Carbs: 4g Fat: 29g Protein: 8g

Servings: 8

Cooking: 2-3 hours

Ingredients:

- ½ C. coconut flour
- ½ C. melted butter
- ½ C. whipping cream
- ½ tsp. xanthan gum
- 1 ½ C. almond flour
- 2 eggs
- 2 tbsp. lemon juice
- 2 tsp. baking powder
- 3 tbsp. swerve sweetener
- Zest of 2 lemons

Topping:

- ½ C. boiling water
- 2 tbsp. lemon juice
- 2 tbsp. melted butter
- 3 tbsp. swerve sweetener

Diet *Preparation:*

1. Combine xanthan gum, baking powder, sweetener, and flours together.

2. Whisk egg, lemon juice and zest, whipping cream, and butter together.

3. Mix dry and wet components together and pour mixture into your greased slowcooker.

4. For topping, combine all topping components till incorporated and spread over top of cake mixture.

5. Set to cook on high 2-3 hours.

6. Serve warm with whipped cream and fresh fruit!

Keto Chocolate Cake

Calories: 357 Carbs: 5g Fat: 26g Protein: 13g

Servings: 6-7

Cooking: 2 ½ hours

Ingredients:

- ¼ tsp. salt
- ½ C. cocoa powder
- ½ C. Swerve
- ¾ tsp. vanilla extract
- 1 ½ tsp. baking powder
- 1 C. + 2 tbsp. almond flour
- 1/3 C. sugar-free chocolate chips
- 2/3 C. unsweetened almond milk
- 3 eggs
- 3 tbsp. whey protein powder
- 6 tbsp. melted butter

Preparation:

1. Grease slowcooker.

2. Mix salt, baking powder, protein powder, cocoa powder, sweetener, and almond flour together.

3. Mix in vanilla, almond milk, eggs, and butter. Fold in chocolate chips.

4. Pour into slowcooker.

5. Set to cook on low 2 ½ hours.

6. Let cool and then slice into pieces.

Blueberry Lemon Custard Cake

Calories: 375 Carbs: 4g Fat: 27g Protein: 14g

Servings: 8-9

Cooking: 3 hours

Ingredients:

- ½ C. sweetener of choice
- ½ C. coconut flour
- ½ C. fresh blueberries
- ½ tsp. salt
- 1 tsp. lemon stevia
- 1/3 C. lemon juice
- 2 C. light cream
- 2 tsp. lemon zest
- 6 separated eggs

Preparation:

1. Add egg whites to a stand mixer, whipping till soft peaks are made.

2. Whisk yolks with remaining ingredients minus blueberries. Fold in egg whites.

3. Grease slowcooker and pour in batter. Sprinkle with blueberries.

4. Set to cook on low 3 hours.

5. Allow to cook at least 1 hour and then chill at least 2 hours or overnight.

6. Serve ice cold with sugar-free whipped cream!

Almond Carrot Cake

Calories: 268 Carbs: 6g Fat: 21g Protein: 6g

Servings: 8

Cooking: 2 hours

Ingredients:

- ¼ C. coconut oil
- ½ C. heavy whipping cream
- ½ C. slivered almonds
- 1 ½ tsp. apple pie spice
- 1 C. almond flour
- 1 C. shredded carrots
- 1 tsp. baking powder
- 3 eggs

Preparation:

1. Grease a cake pan that will fit into the slowcooker.

2. Mix all recipe components with an electric hand mixer, beating till fluffy and incorporated.

3. Pour batter into the pan. With foil, cover pan.

4. Pour 2 cups water into the bottom of slowcooker. Place a trivet over water and carefully place pan onto the trivet.

5. Cook cake for 2 hours on medium heat until done.

6. Take out of the slowcooker and let cool before cutting and
    frosting to eat.

Decadent Chocolate Cake

Calories: 312 Carbs: 3g Fat: 18g Protein: 5g

Servings: 6

Cooking: 2 ½ hours

Ingredients:

- ½ C. unsalted butter
- ½ tsp. baking powder
- ¾ C. almond flour
- ¾ C. cocoa powder
- 1 ½ C. powdered sweetener
- 1 tsp. vanilla extract
- 3 separated eggs

Preparation:

1. Separate eggs. Beat whites with an electric mixer until fluffy. Put to the side.

2. Then beat yolks till smooth and put to the side.

3. Combine baking powder, cocoa powder, and flour. Beat butter and powdered sweetener in a separate bowl until creamy.

4. Add egg whites to butter mixture. Then beat in egg yolks with a hand mixer. Add vanilla and incorporate well.

5. Slowly pour in almond flour mixture to egg mixture, folding well after each new addition.

6. With parchment paper, line a cake pan. Grease with butter. Pour batter into prepared pan.

7. Gently place pan into the slowcooker and cook 2 ½ hours till done in the middle. Indulge without the guilt!

Pumpkin Pie Pudding

Calories: 184 Carbs: 6g Fat: 16g Protein: 3g

Servings: 6

Cooking: 2-3 hours

Ingredients:

- ½ C. heavy whipping cream
- ½ C. heavy whipping cream (for finishing)
- ¾ C. erythritol
- 1 tsp. pumpkin pie spice
- 1 tsp. vanilla extract
- 15 ounces canned pumpkin puree
- 2 eggs

Preparation:

1. Whisk together vanilla extract, pumpkin pie spice, pumpkin puree, erythritol, heavy whipping cream, and eggs.

2. Grease a pan with butter (ensure you get in the corners well!)

3. Pour 1 ½ cups water into your slowcooker Place a trivet over water.

4. Pour batter into pan and gently place pan in a pressure cooker. Cover with a piece of foil.

5. Cook 2 ½ to 3 hours till well combined and custard-like.

6. Before enjoying, chill 6-8 hours.

Banana Nut Bread

Calories: 182 Carbs: 8g Fat: 19g Protein: 11g

Servings: 6

Cooking: 2 hours

Ingredients:

- ¼ C. chopped nuts of choice
- ¼ C. sweetener of choice
- ½ tsp. salt
- 1 ½ tsp. baking soda
- 1/3 C. unsweetened applesauce
- 2 C. low-carb baking mix
- 2 eggs
- 2 tbsp. room temp butter
- 2-3 ripe bananas

Preparation:

1. Combine eggs, applesauce, butter, and sweetener together. Beat with a hand mixer till smooth. Mash bananas and mix in. Add all dry components, incorporating well. Fold in nuts.

2. Grease a pan and pour batter into it. Use a piece of foil to cover.

3. Pour 1 cup of water into the slowcooker, then place a trivet over water and gently place pan onto the trivet.

4. Cook 2 hours till bread is done in the middle. Let cool to room temp before eating.

Conclusion

Congratulations on finishing *The Slowcooker Guide to Keto Diet*!

With the conclusion of this cookbook, you are now more than prepared to journey into the ketogenic diet, and all of its potential to ensure your health of your best self! Plus, you have the convenience of the slowcooker on your side, assisting you in kicking unhealthy temptations out the door.

I hope that the entirety of this cookbook was informative and more valuable than that of other ketogenic cookbooks you have come across. While the ketogenic diet may not be everyone, you never know until you give it a good old-fashioned try! As you have read, there are plenty of delicious and easy-to-make recipes that you can make with the little to no effort, thanks to a highly underestimated kitchen appliance.

Let's face it; being healthy in today's world is much easier said than done, which is why I thrive on the creation of recipe books just like this one! While there are plenty of excuses that can be made regarding the level of health we live by, there are also various ways that we can defeat temptation and stop the process of fueling our bodies with garbage.

I challenge you to begin putting this array of ketogenic recipes to work for you starting *today*. What are you waiting for?

Before I leave you to venture into the ketogenic world for yourself, it would be much appreciated if you could leave a review on Amazon if you found this book valuable, useful, and/or fun to read in any way! Thank you!

9 781720 570110